Is This Really My Child?

Dr. Cathrin Olsen N.D., R.N.

Disclaimer

This book is intended as an informational guide. The approaches and techniques described herein are intended to be used for educational purposes only. They are not intended to be used as medical advice. The author and publisher cannot assume responsibility for the implementation of all of the material or the consequences of its use.

National Library of Canada Cataloguing in Publication Data

A cataloguing record for this book that includes the U.S. Library of Congress Classification number, the Library of Congress Call number and the Dewey Decimal cataloguing code is available from the National Library of Canada. The complete cataloguing record can be obtained from the National Library's online database at: www.nlc-bnc.ca/amicus/index-e.html

ISBN 1-4120-1577-4

TRAFFORD

This book was published on-demand in cooperation with Trafford Publishing.
On-demand publishing is a unique process and service of making a book available for retail sale to the public taking advantage of on-demand manufacturing and Internet marketing. On-demand publishing includes promotions, retail sales, manufacturing, order fulfilment, accounting and collecting royalties on behalf of the author.

Suite 6E, 2333 Government St., Victoria, B.C. V8T 4P4, CANADA
Phone   250-383-6864   Toll-free   1-888-232-4444 (Canada & US)
Fax   250-383-6804   E-mail   sales@trafford.com
Web site   www.trafford.com TRAFFORD PUBLISHING IS A DIVISION OF
                              TRAFFORD HOLDINGS LTD.
Trafford Catalogue #03-1954   www.trafford.com/robots/03-1954.html

10   9   8   7   6   5   4   3   2

Do you see your child?

	Yes	No
Does your child not seem to hear what you are saying?	☐	☐
Is your child clumsy?	☐	☐
Is your child fine one minute and out of control the next?	☐	☐
Does your child chew on clothes?	☐	☐
Is your child unresponsive to discipline?	☐	☐
Does your child run instead of walk, is in constant motion?	☐	☐
Does your child have mood swings?	☐	☐

Do you see your child?

	Yes	No
Is your child sad and listless?	☐	☐
Is your child loud, interruptive?	☐	☐
Is your child persistent and has a low frustration level?	☐	☐
Does your child have difficulty sleeping, falling asleep?	☐	☐
Does your child have frequent physical complaints? Headaches, ear infections, hives, asthma, stomach aches, constipation, bedwetting, muscle aches?	☐	☐

Acknowledgement

Special thanks goes to many people who helped make this book possible. Debbie Lavage, Lance Humphrey for proof reading and suggestions. Jeannie Stange for being my sounding board. My mother for encouraging my independence. My children for inspiring me to write.

The Information provided to you in this book will address the relationship between certain food items, behavior and physical ailments.

Step One is set up to give you almost immediate relief from your ordeal and provide you a way to see the light at the end of the tunnel.

I will explain specific food sensitivities, which foods to avoid and why. We will then move on to the "boundaries, empathy, consistency, love and laughter approach (BECLL) ," which will give you an innovative new way of interacting with your children and provide you with guidelines to make positive changes to your relationship with them. The goal is to have one good day, then two good days and then three, and so on. Slow and consistent progress is the key.

In *Step Two* you will reintroduce certain foods to your child's diet and you will be able to tell if your child has any food sensitivity to them. Furthermore, we will discuss food combinations and easy-to-follow guidelines for specific food choices to keep your child happy and content. Last, but not least, we will discuss environmental culprits and how they may cause reactions. I will take you through this process, step by step. This will be fun; you will see. You will be motivated.

You will be able to see results fast, and your stress level will go down. ☺

Contents at a glance

Contents at a glance

Contents at a glance

CONCLUSION

A note from the Author
Membership information

*This book is dedicated to
Mark, my husband
with love and admiration*

Five a.m. in the morning and I am sitting on the top of the steps crying. The boy is awake—already. He went to bed at 10:30 p.m. and he is awake. What is wrong with this child? What is wrong with me? It must be the genes. His sister did stuff like this too; she grew out of it, but she is still difficult. She is 14 now. It's genetic; I know it is my fault. It is my genes. What am I doing wrong? I don't have a handle on it—on anything; I just react all day long. I can't keep up with him. He is all over the place, constantly running, into everything, he never stops and is so anxious. He is driving me crazy. I am so very tired. I just want a few minutes for me. I just don't like him, I don't like my life, I don't like anything. How can it be? Oh God, I feel so guilty, so bad. I am going to lose my mind, I know it. How can this beautiful four-year-old boy with those big brown eyes be _such a disaster? When is this going to end? I don't like him! Now I feel really bad for even thinking that._

How can you not like your own child? It's me, all my fault.

I am a horrible mother.

I can't do this anymore.

That was me two years ago. I had this beautiful four year old baby boy who was persistent, nonstop, never slept, nervous, broke everything in sight, climbed on everything (especially things that should not be climbed on), and pitched temper tantrums.

My son, Liam is seven years old now.

A delightful thoughtful, kind and gentle, smiling child. He sleeps well, loves to play, is eager to please, calm, in control, happy and energetic. Temperamentally he is still persistent, focused and high strung. However, these traits are much easier to channel into positive areas.

What brought on the change?

In my research I found a strong correlation between food, vitamins and behavior. I had been a RN for many years and was in the process of getting my doctorate in Naturology. I had worked in the psychiatric field and just felt that there had to be another way, other than drugs, to deal with my child and other children like him.

Medication use

I purposely am not addressing the use of Ritalin or medications similar to Ritalin. My program is an approach for restoring optimal health with some behavior modification.

A Lifestyle not a diet!

Please contact your medical provider for medication use.

I believe that your child will benefit greatly from my approach. You will notice behavioral changes in your child and he or she will be happier, calmer and more content. I think that you, as a parent, have choices and the responsibility and the right to make appropriate decisions for your child's wellbeing. Therefore, I strongly encourage you to follow up with your medical doctor for any questions on medication use.

Research all your choices, including mine. You also may want to visit my website at *www.ADDnomore.com* for in-depth information on medication use and side effects.

I have had clients take their children entirely off medication after adapting my approach. Other clients were able to decrease their children's medications considerably. Ritalin and similar medications do have significant side effects. Research has revealed long-standing health problems related to the use of Ritalin and similar medications.

Vitamins

I am not advocating vitamins for children.

It is important for children to receive proper nutrients and minerals through their day-to-day food intake.

We need to teach our children proper eating habits and awareness of their bodies' needs.

In some instances, a child's health may seem to indicate a need for supplemental vitamin or mineral use. A professional consultant should first make a thorough assessment of your child.

You are the ONE!!

I would like to address one important area prior to getting started.

I know you are tired and might feel that you don't have the strength to continue on, or to try something else, something new. I have good news and bad news for you. The bad news is that no one, and I mean no one, will be able to bring harmony and tranquility into your life—except you!

You can take your kids to a medical doctor, therapist, school counselor, or clergy. You can keep them in day care all day and pick them up late so you don't have to deal with them. You can leave them at their grandparents', aunts', uncles' or other relatives' houses. The list goes on. Yet, every time you are with your child you will continue to have to deal with the physical and emotional aspects of your child. You will have to interact.

The longer you wait, the harder it will become. The more hurtful things you will say and do, the more frustrated you will become.

Your family will fall apart.

You are the only one, who can "fix" this. You are the only one who knows your child and who loves him or her so much that you put up with all the frustration and pain. You are the only one who sees that your child is suffering and desperately wants to succeed and be happy. I feel for you, but you are the one—the only one.

The good news is that I feel very confident that you will see great progress in a very short time. My approach is easy to follow and is encouraging. It is not a diet, but a New Lifestyle.

This lifestyle is designed for the entire family and will be beneficial to everyone.

You will start feeling in control and have hope.

Feeling sane—what a concept!

And who knows? You may find that your child is a lot more like you, than different from you. ☺

Let's get started!

Step One

I will discuss food changes and behavior. You will be able to start immediately and will see the light at the end of the tunnel.

Promise!!!! Easy and fast. The more you adopt the concept of this approach, the faster you will see results.

All food should be natural.

This means that you need to use butter instead of margarine, regular Ranch dressing instead of non-fat, regular cheese instead of low fat. You are wondering about the fat?

Your body is able to metabolize fat much better than heaps of non-natural chemicals, food coloring, and preservatives. I believe that one of the reasons people are overweight, is not the fat they eat, but the amount of chemicals their bodies accumulate by making the wrong food choices.

The weight is a consequence of the body's inability to get rid of the chemicals within the food.

Suzanne Lawton, ND, states at her website: *www.Naturpathyonline.com* that "Margarine adheres to the walls of the blood vessels in your body—thick plastic coating that has been associated with worsening aspects of atherosclerosis. Our bodies have a substance called butyric acid, which helps break down butter. The next time you go to the store look at the ingredients of low fat dressing and compare to the regular dressing. You will notice a lot more ingredients that do not sound natural."

If you can't pronounce it, don't eat it!!!!

Sodas are a No-No.

Do you know that Pepsi or Coke is used to clear out clogged feeding tubes for patients? The acid is so strong in sodas that it eats through the debris. Imagine what your stomach looks like after drinking this, day in and day out. Now imagine your child's stomach.

You are thinking "but juices are fine, the ones in a box." Right? Wrong!

Read the label! Ingredients are sugar water and artificial flavoring.

Make your own soda, by adding pear or pineapple juice to a little bit of sparkling water.

You just made your own healthy refreshing soda. ☺

Faucet water

No matter where you live in the U.S., you should not drink faucet water. Buy bottled water or a purifier. A distiller is by far the best method. Encourage your child to drink more water; most children do not drink enough fluids any-way. Water is good for you.

Add a slice of lemon or lime and a fresh mint leaf. Make it fancy. Children love this.

Ice cream

Ice cream advertised as "natu-ral" does not mean it is 100% natural. Double-check the in-gredients. Make sure there are no dyes or artificial flavor like vanillin. Vanillin is not Va-nilla. Big difference!

Vanilla is the only natural form of flavoring, all others are artificial replicas.

Candy

Candy is a favorite of children everywhere.

As you become more aware, you will notice that almost all candy has to be eliminated from your child's diet; because most candy contains dyes and artificial coloring.

Believe it or not chocolate bars are better then any colored candies or gum.

You can make your own candy; it is not difficult and is fun to prepare with your child. (I have listed recipes in the back of the book). In time your child will be able to tolerate a few pieces of candy here and there and will be able to process a few no-no items on occasion.

Substitute, do not deprive!

Sugar

Sugar is used in many foods, but in itself it is not the culprit. Moderation, of course, is the key to everything. If you look closely, you will notice that in addition to the sugar your child may have ingested a cherry lollipop and an orange Popsicle. Yes, a large amount of sugar; however, there are much more dyes and artificial flavors than anything else. Again, balance is incorporated and you must use your own judgment. Recognize the different names for sugar: corn syrup, corn sweetener, fructose, sucrose, dextrose or glucose. Add natural sweeteners instead of sugar such as banana, honey or figs.

Never use artificial sweeteners. Aspartame, an artificial sweetener, has been linked to dozens of conditions such as increased appetite, migraines or anxiety. Unrefined sugar is a natural food.

Use it in moderation.

*You know your child better
than anyone.*

Be inventive...use moderation.

Milk

Throughout history, children have always been encouraged to drink milk. I, for one, am against large amounts of milk consumption by children. Milk has been linked to repeated ear infections, sinus infections, digestive disorders and bedwetting. Repeated coughs and asthma attacks are also associated with milk consumption. Many people lack the enzymes needed to digest cow milk. Just compare the size of a calf to a human baby. The proteins are designed for a calf.

There are many other ways to include proper nutrients in your child's diet, such as eating healthy, natural, non-processed foods and using organic milk, which contains no hormones.

If your child drinks milk and has a bedwetting problem, try to limit milk drinking to no later than 6 p.m. and then slowly move the time back so that the child will eventually end up with only one glass of milk in the morning, preferably just with cereal. At the same time, you are restricting your child's milk drinking to earlier and earlier in the day, start giving your child soy milk with cereal in the morning.

They will not notice the difference.

You can buy soy milk in the regular grocery store and should try the chocolate soy milk or vanilla—really good! If you choose to continue the use of regular milk, you should buy the organic cow milk.

Organic cow milk is derived from cows that have not been injected with hormones or antibiotics and have not been fed food, that has been treated with pesticides.

Meat

Buy naturally grown meats, preferably free range.

Like the organic milk, organic meat is free of antibiotics, added hormones, and other hormones and drugs. The animals used for organic meat graze freely and are considered "free range." The bovine human growth hormone is never used in "free range" meat. For example, mad cow disease derives from feeding cattle ground-up carcasses of the same species, which develops the bovine spongiform encephalopathy, which destroys the central nervous system and brain of humans.

Just think about the implications of feeding non-meat-eating animals ground up dead particles of their kind. There is something really wrong with this!!!!

Try to buy chicken, beef, lamb, and pork that have been processed naturally.

Purchase free-range, natural eggs. (Which means the chicken lived in a natural environment and laid eggs the old-fashioned way).

Food dyes and food coloring

Food coloring, food dyes, synthetic colors, artificial colors, and specific preservatives are a no-no. Nothing natural is in these items. Blue ketchup? Green French fries?

How can we expect our children to digest food coloring and dyes? Jane Hersey writes in her book *Why can't my child behave?* "Today most colorings are created from petroleum, the source for gasoline, kerosene, and asphalt, but they are often still referred to us as coal-tar dyes. Food dyes are known to be cancer causing chemicals."

Need I say more?

You will see them written in many different ways.

Starting with FD&C and D&C followed by:

Yellow No. 5,6,10

Red 3,7,22,27,28,30,33,40

Blue 1,2

Green 3

Start reading the labels!

You will notice that even shampoo or body lotion have dyes added.

Your skin is the largest organ of your body and absorbs substances and chemicals just like your lungs or stomach. Switch to another, healthier brand.

Start reading labels!!!

In no time will you know which items you can buy. It is easier to shop at the health food store and often you will obtain great items for less money than at the supermarket.

Buy bulk for items such as pastas, flours, soup mixes, cereal, oatmeal, rice or granola.

There are many different preservatives;

I am most concerned with three specific preservatives. These are antioxidant preservatives and are petroleum based.

Yes, they are made from petroleum and we eat them!!!

Day in and day out our bodies have to digest these poisons.

They seem to cause the most havoc in the brain and need to be totally eliminated from your child's diet, and, if you like, from yours too. You as an adult can benefit greatly.

They are:

BHA:

Butylated Hydroxyanisole

BTA:

Butylated Hydrooxytoluene

TBHQ:

Tertiary Buytylhydroquinone

Most restaurant oils used for deep frying are preserved with TBHQ.

Food and Behavior

I consider Dr. Ben Feingold to be the pioneer in recognizing the correlation between food and behavior. I have incorporated his philosophy and guidelines within my book.

Dr. Feingold established *The Feingold Program*, a non profit organization.

Dr. Ben Feingold was a pediatrician in California. He eventually specialized in child allergies.

According to the *Feingold Association Handbook:* "In 1965 Dr. Feingold began observations of the link between certain foods and additives and their effect on some individual's behavior and ability to learn. Dr. Feingold presented his findings to the American Medical Association in June 1973; he called upon the scientific community to research and test his hypothesis. But the science of the biochemical basis for behavior was and still is in its infancy and Dr. Feingold knew it would be decades before details of the relationship between foods and behavior would be fully understood."

Dr. Feingold believed his most important responsibility as a clinician was the obligation to offer practical assistance to the troubled patient.

He developed a program that could dramatically help more than half of the children and adults he saw, a program that was relatively simple to use and inexpensive. It presented no harmful side effects.

I have incorporated these aspects within my program.

The Feingold Program focuses on educating the public about the relationship between certain food additives and salicylates and their effect on behavior and learning.

The Feingold Program outlines completed research on food items that are produced in specific geographical areas and eliminates the need for users of his program to do most of the footwork. You can become a member for a small one-time fee and receive much helpful information from them.

Chapter I

Salicylates

Pronounced:
Suh'lis'uh'lates

Salicylates are natural substances in certain foods. Plants make salicylates to protect themselves from bacteria by natural predators. The plant increases production of salicylates when threatened and sends messages to nearby plants to do the same.

Salicylates appear to exist as a natural preservative or insecticide that protects the plant and extends its life span.

Many scientists worldwide have researched natural salicylates in foods and how they affect behavior. *The Journal of the American Dietetic Association Vol. 85:8* (1985) discussed the work of Anne Swain and others in Australia in the mid 1980's who demonstrated the extent to which Salicylate is present in food. Aspirin is the most well known salicylate and aspirin sensitivity is recognized throughout the world.

Nothing is wrong with food items which contain Salicylates; in fact they are exceptionally good for your health.

Some people, however, are sensitive to them. They can cause adverse reactions and produce anything from asthma to violent tempers. Each person can react differently to foods containing salicylates. The actual cause of why some people are salicyate sensitive is still a mystery.

It is also not known why some people are sensitive to one item, but not to another. Much research has been done, but at this time too little is known about salicylate sensitivity. The research done at Kaiser-Permanente Medical Center in San Francisco demonstrated a link between food dyes, aspirin and some foods.

The most peculiar thing is that the reaction to these items could vary from patient to patient. Some items would bring about a physical reaction such as hives or rash and others a decrease in learning or a violent outburst.

Dr. Feingold pioneered the use of the *elimination process technique*, which assists people in determining which Salicylates affect their general health, behavior, or learning ability.

This method removes all the foods containing Salicylate and reintroduces them one by one into the diet. It is a process of elimination.

These food items contain natural Salicylates and need to be eliminated from your child's diet. You need to stop using these food items alto-gether at the same time:

Almonds   **Grapes**
Coffee   **Raisin**
Peaches   **Tangerine**
Apples   **Cherries**
Cucumber   **Nectarines**
Pickles   **Tea**
Peppers   **Cloves**
Apricot   **Oranges**
Currants   **Tomato**
Plums   **Oil of Win-**
Prunes   **tergreen**
All Berries

Any form of these items; fresh, frozen, juiced, dried or canned.

For example: no apple juice, apple sauce, apple pie, apple cider, fresh apples, dried apples, or trail mix with apple pieces.

Don't panic.

I know these are great food items and you are saying, "I can't do this!!! That is all we eat." Remember, these items will be reintroduced one by one in *Step Two*.

Some people are sensitive to strawberries, but can eat tomatoes without any problems. It is difficult to know which item is a problem—especially since a child can consume strawberries, tomatoes, pickles, and apple juice all in one day.

Therefore, we clean up the body by taking all the items

out of the equation in *Step One*.

Then in *Step Two*, we reintroduce these items one by one.

I want to tell you an actual story, just to make my point.

We went to a picnic on 4th July weekend and ate the usual hot dogs and hamburgers. My husband felt that we should let our son have fun and not worry about the ingredients of hot dogs: food coloring, chemicals and dyes.

Only for today.

"Oh, let him have fun".

I agreed, thinking one day would not make a difference.

We were so wrong!!!!

So very wrong!

The next day our son was running into things, falling down, biting his brother, chewing on his clothes, had two temper tantrums, would not take a nap, was constantly moving about, crying, anxious, and was continuously saying he was hungry.

Then, to top it off, wet the bed after having a horrible time going to sleep.

We are still learning.

Nothing is worth seeing him in such agony. Forget about the "Oh, let him have fun."

It is not fun!!!!!

Buy soy hotdogs and hamburgers. Drink papaya, mango, or pear juice with sparkling water, and you will still have fun. ☺

Long-term fun.

More than one day. No regrets.

Really, it is not worth it.

The faster you succeed in following the guidelines, the faster you will see results.

You will remain in *Step One* for four to six weeks for your child, or as long as is needed to feel good and realize progress. Even if you have to re-lax and enjoy the calmness, don't get fixated on four to six weeks.

That is just an estimate.

I took longer. I was so tired and drained I did not want to chance the negative affects of salicylates again.

I needed more time, which was not a problem.

This program is for you and you make the decision. OK? ☺

Now you are wondering what you can eat, and drink, right?

Believe it or not you still have a lot of choices.

They include, but are not lim-ited to:

Artichokes	Beef
Asparagus	Beets
Avocados	Biscuits
Bagels	Bread
Bamboo	Broccoli
Banana	Butter
Barley	Cabbage
Beans	Cake

Candy	Flour
Cantaloupe	Garlic
Carrots	Gelatin
Cashew	Grains
Nuts	Granola
Celery	Grapefruit
Cereal	Hamburger
Cheese	Honey
Chicken	Honeydew
Chinese	Hot dogs
Veggies	Ice cream
Chips	Jam & jelly
Chives	Kiwi
Cocoa	Lamb
Chocolate	Lemon &
Coconut	Lime
Cookies	Lettuce
Corn	Lobster
Cornmeal	Macaroni
Crabmeat	Mango
Crackers	Mayonnaise
Cream	Milk
Cream	Molasses
Cheese	Muffins
Dates	Mushroom
Eggs	Mustard
Eggplant	Noodles
English	Oatmeal
Muffins	Olives
Figs	Oates

Olive oil
Onion
Pancakes
Papaya
Pasta
Peanuts
Peanut but-
ter
Pears
Peas
Pecan
Pepper
Pie
Pineapple
Pistachio
Pita bread
Pomegran-
ate
Popcorn
Pork
Potatoes
Pretzel
Pudding
Pumpkin
Radishes
Roast beef
Rice
Rice cakes
Rolls
Salad

Salad
dressing
Salmon
Salt
Sausage
Scallion
Seafood
Seeds
Sherbet
Shortening
Shrimp
Soda
Sorbet
Soy sauce
Soup
Sour cream
Spinach
Squash
Steak
String-
beans
Sugar
Sweet-
potatoes
Syrup
Toast
Tuna
Turkey
Veal

Vegetable oil
Vinegar
Waffles
Walnuts
Water-chestnuts

Watercress
Watermelon
Yams
Yeast
Yogurt
Zucchini

See—lots of food to eat!

Plan on taking a little bit longer to learn to look at labels and to revise your shopping list. In no time at all will you have mastered this. Trust me.

I found going to the health food store solves a lot of problems and some foods are also cheaper. For example, cereal is hard to buy at the regular store, since most contain either food coloring or dyes.

A health food store has a great variety of organic cereal, organic snacks and they taste good too. You can also buy in bulk.

Chapter I

Now—don't stress out. Take your time.

Be kind to yourself ☺.

Step One – Behavior

Some children in our society are considered "difficult." Society has labeled them and forgotten that under all the labeling a young person exists. Often a very unhappy person, consumed with frustration.

It is your job as a parent to protect and nurture this child. I am giving you tools to do so. You have to see which particular ones work and choose the ones for you. You may find that all of them work; you may find that only one or two work for your particular situation.

I don't like labeling. I believe in channeling these "difficult" children in the right direction.

By using their abundance of energy in a positive light, they will become wonderful adults, able to contribute to society. I find most of these kids are temperamentally difficult, which means they are very determined, high strung, energetic, insightful, goal oriented, feisty, opinionated and passionate. Now let's compare this list of attributes to successful people in this world.

Surprise, surprise—they have the same attributes!!!!

Stanley Turecki, M.D., discusses in his book *The difficult Child*, "that of course not all of our children can become famous, but who knows what greatness lies ahead for our children. We should always treat our children with kindness and love, respect them, foster his or her abilities and always remember he or she is an individual."

Turecki tells a story of a great man who was thought of as a horrible, bad child in his youth.

The story goes:

"Then there is a story of a most difficult child, a redheaded swaggerer who was disobedient and always in trouble, who was constantly in motion, always jumping up and down, leaping, rushing around and falling and hurting himself. The words 'hyperactive and difficult' were both used to describe him. He was thought to be 'dull' intellectually, prone to frequent colds and skin rashes, an uncoordinated weakling with a speech impediment whose school records, one of the lowest in his class, reflected a history of misconduct and failure.

The boy's name?

Winston Spencer Churchill."

Sir Winston Spencer Churchill 1874-1965, was the Prime Minister of the United Kingdom in World War II.

He was also a noted speaker, author, painter, soldier and war reporter.

Chapter I

In 1953 he won the Nobel Prize for Literature.

Need I say more?

BECLL Approach

Boundaries, Empathy, Consistency, Love and Laughter Approach.

The *BECLL Approach* came about as I was contemplating the most important attributes used by highly effective parents. Throughout my research I realized that highly effective parents with happy and well adjusted children have one common denominator:

The *BECLL Approach,* which stands for boundaries, empathy, consistency, love and laughter.

Boundaries

Boundaries are an essential tool for all children. Boundaries allow the child to grow and feel secure and nurtured within the realm of expectations. Staying within the boundaries increases the child's self esteem and self worth. Furthermore, it decreases power struggles between the child and parents.

You should set boundaries which you as a parent can abide by and feel comfortable with.

Don't set your goals too high, or you run the risk of becoming frustrated when the goals aren't met. Establish basic boundaries.

- Have a set bedtime
- Have a set meal time
- Be clear on TV programs allowed
- Be clear on rules for snacks

- Be clear on basic discipline issues

Empathy

Empathy is the ability to feel emotional for another person without actually sharing that person's experiences. It is the ability to appreciate another's suffering.

Acknowledge your child's feelings even though you may not be able to understand them or relate to them. Show your child that you care about his or her feelings and allow individuality. This does not mean that you will agree with them, by any means. You have to be emotionally removed and not take things personally. Stay with the issue at hand and do not worry about the motives of the child. This, of course is easier said than done. You might not be able to instantly achieve this detachment and calmness. Yet, make a firm but kind statement.

Be patient and give it time.

Here are a few examples:

No-no: "Why do you always do this to me when it is time to go to bed?"

Instead, say: "I understand that some nights are hard for you to go to bed and sleep."

No-no: "Let it go! I can't believe you are acting like this! It drives me crazy!"

Instead, say: "I know it is hard for you to let something go and give it up when you really want something."

No-no: "Stop screaming and yelling so loudly."

Instead, say: "I know you have a loud voice, but...."

No-no: "I said, let's go! How many times do I have to tell you?"

Instead, say: "I know it is hard for you to change what

you are doing. I will give you two minutes to get ready."

By acknowledging your child's behavior you will provide empathy and at the same time redirect your child to the appropriate behavioral path.

Another example would be:

"I know you are overwhelmed by all the things you need to get done before you can watch cartoons. I understand; I can help you. What would you like to do first: Make your bed or get dressed?"

You will find that your child will react favorably to this and you will see results without the usual power struggles and negative domino effect.

Your attitude is the key; you have to remain calm and detached. Stop thinking, "Why is he or she doing this to me?"

Your child is not doing this to you! ☺

Consistency

Consistency is difficult but most important. Being consistent with a child is acting or conducting yourself in the same manner in every circumstance to arrive at a desirable outcome in every situation.

The same, over and over again.

Setting boundaries and providing empathy are great tools, but they have little bearing if they are not used the same way time after time.

It is very challenging to be consistent. I understand you are tired. Sometimes you feel that if you give in now, that at least you will have a few minutes of peace. You are correct in that; however, the price you pay in a later conflict will be tenfold for not being consistent. Your child will be persistent and as the persisting increases, so will the temper tantrums.

This is *The Golden Rule* of the BECLL Approach to child discipline.

You have to stay firm and consistent; you have to.

Put a note on the refrigerator!!!!!

Keep reminding yourself.

Be consistent.

Love

Love is the expression of one's affection. Show your child your love.

Be kind and gentle to your children when they cannot be kind to themselves. Love them when they do not love themselves.

Play with him or her for fifteen minutes a day. Give each child individual time. Sit with him or her, and ask how the day went, how they feel. Just listening will make your child feel important. During this special time do not cook, talk on the phone, write bills or answer emails.

You are busy and your day is full....and...and....and...STOP!

Just give your child fifteen minutes a day of undivided attention.

By focusing on the good, your child will step up to the plate and will want to receive praise from you. Don't say negative remarks out loud. Stop being sarcastic or cynical. Children do not respond well to sarcasm.

Do not use "always" or "never."

It is impossible to be always a pain, always bad, always horrible or never right, never perfect, never ok.

Try not to use these words.

If you don't have anything nice to say, don't say anything at all.

It will take time to change, but you will. Be kind to yourself.

You can change. Your child can change. Just do it. Let the old ways go.

Here are a few ideas for you

- Give one compliment a day

- Focus on the positive attribute

- Say "I love you."

- Say "I am proud of you."

- Say "I like when you do this."

- Play Legos or Barbie on the floor for fifteen minutes.

- Give a kiss, a hug.

Stay within your set boundaries, give empathy, be consistent and show love.

Try these approaches:

- You should try to leave social gatherings while your child is still happy and not burned out or tired.

- Leave while your child is still in high spirits, happy and having fun.

- Leave the pool at 2 p.m. instead of 4 p.m.

- Leave the amusement park an hour early so that you can avoid the long exit lines.

- Don't be last person to leave the birthday party, leave while everyone is still happy and having fun.

- Don't wait until it turns into a disaster or another power struggle.

- Leave before your child has a *meltdown* !!!!

Laughter

The last, but certainly not least, is laughter.

Find something your child and you can laugh about. It is not necessary to spend money. Amusement parks are too stimulating for a difficult child anyway. Amusement parks inevitably lead to power struggles, which always make for a horrible day. I have been twice to an amusement park and my children range from seven to seventeen years of age.

Trust me: Never again! ☺

Laughing every day is easier said than done. We want to focus on the positive, so we will make "Happy times and Happy thoughts."

To build positive communication between you and your children, you have to develop happy memories you share with them, by doing funny and silly things.

Your mood will get better and so will your child's. Pretend you are happy and content and eventually you will feel happy and content.

Here are a few examples:

- Sing in the car; change the words to a familiar tune

- Skip with your child down the sidewalk

- Jump rope

- Make funny faces

- Blow bubbles

- Distort your face

- Make weird sounds

- Try to have fun

- Watch less TV

You have now established the principles of *Step One.*

Implement these ideas, as best as you can. The closer you can remain within the guidelines the faster you will see results. Don't get disheartened if you are unable to make these changes fast or slip back to the old methods. Be kind, loving and patient to yourself and your family. Learn how to notice small changes in you child. Remember, it did not take your child just two weeks to get this way. You will have to motivate your child and be happy for every small change you and your child will achieve.

Small steps will get you there.☺

Is this program working for your child?

Is this program working for your child? Check if your child is displaying any changes in his or her behavior. Are you noticing anything different? No matter how small?

Is your child:

- ✓ Able to sit at the dinner table without getting up
- ✓ Able to look at you when talked to
- ✓ Able to follow directions a little bit better
- ✓ Able to refocus
- ✓ Able to finish more homework at a time
- ✓ Able to have fun with friends without an argument
- ✓ Able to last 3 hours without a temper tantrum
- ✓ Able to go to sleep

- ✓ Throwing or breaking things less
- ✓ Chewing on clothes less
- ✓ Able to be more patient
- ✓ Experiencing fewer mood swings
- ✓ Responding to discipline
- ✓ Walking instead of running
- ✓ Less loud
- ✓ Able to finish more of a project then before
- ✓ Able to want a kiss or a hug

Remain in *Step One* for four to six weeks. Get comfortable with the process. Then we will move on to Step Two. Introducing more alternatives for food choices, reintroducing salicylates and various other issues. You can do this. ☺

I feel so different about my son

My son is a changed boy after seven weeks of starting this program.

I was so overwhelmed, that I required two weeks merely to get the food items correct without dye and coloring. Concentrating on removing the salicylates from the diet was a major effort. I was afraid to reintroduce them. I thought it was almost not worth it, and I was enjoying the peace and my happy child.

How would I explain to my child that he couldn't have apples, strawberries and grapes or oranges?

I sat at the kitchen table with him and explained how I wanted to try something new with him and that I thought that a lot of his behavior was not his fault and I told him that.

You should have seen his face!!!!

For the first time he believed he was no longer responsible for his actions. His face lit up, he really loved that idea.

This is the way to go! I was proud of myself. I found a way for him to agree to eliminate the salicylates, dyes and food coloring and at the same time avoided a power struggle. A week later he told everyone that he couldn't eat this or that item because it hurt his head and made him do crazy things. Quicker than I could have ever imagined he ended up telling me that he could no longer eat grapes and peaches, because they were hurting his head.

Liam can't read yet; however, he would clarify if he could eat an item.

"Can I eat this, Mommy? Is this good for me?" Liam was so very proud of himself. He was actually having fun. I real-

ized that not only did I want him to have a good day; he wanted to have a great day, too. His demeanor changed. He is lovable. He kisses me all the time and wants to be hugged. He is able to sit and watch a movie or watch an entire soccer game sitting on my lap. He is able to follow a storyline in a book; discuss the day's events; and is kind and compassionate to his friends, brother, sisters, our dog.

I have calmed down, too. I am able to take a shower and not wonder where he is, if he is hanging out of the window or climbing the kitchen cabinets. A car ride to and from school is now calm and enjoyable.

I actually like him ☺ Going to the park is fun. Tantrums are almost nonexistent. He remains persistent, but the great thing is, once I show him empathy and say, "I know this is hard, I understand," he lets go, we can make the transition, *and the day remains great. I can breathe; I can have a calm day.*

More than anything. I like my child. I no longer feel like such a failure.

Step Two

At this point you have been in *Step One* for four to six weeks, maybe longer—no worries!!! ☺

Your child should be acting a little different: *good* different.

Noticeable and significant changes have occurred, right?

Great, so we will continue with *Step Two*.

Initially in *Step Two*, I will show you how to reintroduce foods with salicylates into your daily regimen and what signs to watch out for. I will also show you what to do if your child has a reaction to reintroduced salicylate items. Furthermore, I will discuss food variation and food combinations to promote health and natural good habits.

I will touch on environmental culprits and how they can affect your child's behavior.

Salicylates

Before you begin reintroduction of food items, you need to know a few facts and what to look out for.

You should have noticed the correlation between what your child eats and how he or she behaves.

These are the guidelines:

- Reintroduce only one salicylate fruit or vegetable at a time.

- Wait three to four days before introducing another one.

- Buy organic or locally grown produce; fresh is the best.

- Notice that your child may have sensitivity to some food types, apples for instance, but not others, like oranges.

- Reaction to newly indicated foods may vary as well. Your child may tolerate red apples, for example, but not green apples.

- Salicylate levels in foods may vary depending on whether they are cooked, raw, or frozen and which area in the country you live.

- Raw, peeled foods seem to be better than cooked foods with the skin remaining.

- Be careful with the cumulative effect of salicylates. After introducing a few items you may suddenly notice a reaction, even though your child was fine before. Remove one item, or just simply go back to *Step One*.

You may find in time that your child is able to tolerate a lot of the natural salicylate-containing foods, even though sensitivity was high at the beginning.

Environmental Culprits

Chemicals are all around us.

In the food, in the water, in our homes, and at schools. Most people do not correlate getting sick to their environment. Does your child have frequent colds, coughs or is irritable for no reason? Does your child act like a hypochondriac: always something wrong with him or her? Are there no apparent reasons why he or she is so sickly?

People can get very ill from environmental toxins. Remember the story about Erin Brockovich?

Did you move to a new home, buy new carpet, or paint your child's room? Did the school install new carpet or vinyl flooring? These are valid concerns and you should evaluate your child's environment.

After we had moved into our new house, two out of out five children were always sick.

Nothing really bad, but just not feeling good, swollen lymph nodes, sore throats, headaches, always tired and difficulty falling a sleep.

I found myself not feeling so well either: a constant slight headache, swollen membranes in my nose, just plain irritable.

Suddenly, I realized that our ailments were probably correlated to the products in our new home. New paint, new carpet, new everything. Fumes from the new house were being released. Our new house smells were making us sick!

I invested in an air purifier. This purifier was able to "clean up" the air and remove the toxic fumes at a faster rate than the natural airing out of the house.

I noticed an improvement in our health. Nothing extreme, but the children had more energy. There was less coughing and better sleep patterns. My headaches were gone.

Even though you think the air freshener smells "spring fresh", it is not spring fresh!!!!

You cannot put natural smells into the air with an air freshener. The fragrance is derived by mixing multiple chemicals.

Nothing natural about that!!!!!

Evaluate your choice of your household cleaning supply, too.

Do you use air fresheners, carpet fresheners, dust with products like pledge, and wipe the children's toys with bleach products?

I strongly urge you to investigate these possible culprits within your home. You can purchase air filters and purifiers to accelerate the process. Buy cleaning supplies from a health food store. Otherwise your children have to eliminate these toxins from their little bodies.

Make your life easier. Buy natural products!!!!

How can you tell if your child is having a reaction?

A reaction is much easier to detect in a teenager than in younger children. Try to watch for an undesirable behavior. You can use the list below to evaluate your child's behavior.

Signs of possible reactions to natural salicylate can occur anywhere from one to seventy-two hours after exposure.

It could be a reaction if:

- A healthy snack doesn't help

- Your child is not hearing you

- The problem lasts an entire day

- A nap or rest doesn't help

- A reaction can last up to four or five days

You will need to follow the BECLL Approach in *Step One* as much as possible.

Be kind and compassionate ☺

"Emotionally disengage." This is easier said than done. I realize that, but there will be an end to this, because you know why your child is acting, the way he or she is.

You are in charge! ☺

Here are a few guidelines:

- Maintain the BECLL Approach: Boundaries, Empathy, Consistency,

- Love and Laughter.

- Avoid stressful situations.

- Cancel parties and family gatherings.

- Provide a calm environment.

- Let your child take a soothing bath.

- Encourage drinking lots of water, flushing out the toxins.

- Wait until after the re-action is over to talk about it.

After this is over, sit down with your child, even at a young age; discuss the food as "culprit".

Make sure the child is aware that he or she was not at fault, it was the food to blame. Optimistically discuss how you both will avoid these culprits, in the future.

This is a great learning tool for school age children. No child wants to feel awful. You can teach children to take responsibility for their food intake, even at school.

They will know the negative effects of the food culprits and won't want to act that way in school.

Chapter II

This "reaction" can be very positive and educational for both, you and your child.

One day after we picked up his sister from school, my son was acting out by refusing to follow directions.

I ended up losing my cool and yelled: "Just stop it, stop it now!" I was quite angry and Liam proceeded to cry. Once I calmed down and he stopped crying we started to talk about the situation.

Liam muttered: "...but, but, Mommy, I did not do it, really. the grapes made me do it!"

I had to smile.

We have smart children. ☺

I realized for the first time, in a long long time, that he was just being a normal appropriate, misbehaving child.

Nothing more, nothing less.

Unreal! Typical child behavior!

My child ?!?!?!!

Never in my wildest dreams did I imagine that I would refer to my child's behavior as "typical".

Never did I think I would be so ecstatic over my child's misbehavior. ☺

Make sure that you are aware and tuned in to the fundamental differences of these behaviors and the effects on your child.

Ask yourself: is it basic misbehaving, or is it food related and can not be helped?

Did you know?

For most children the crucial thing is to break the pattern of failure by giving them many opportunities to be successful.

What does the body need?

In this next section I will discuss protein, carbohydrate, and fat and how each one functions and interacts within your body.

Balance and moderation is the key. I will explain why balance is so crucial and show you how to combine the correct nutritional items, to achieve optimal health for your child.

Furthermore, I will list recipes, snack ideas. I will also touch on special events like Halloween and birthday parties.

Protein

A constant supply of protein is required for the body to build tissues and contribute to natural chemical reactions in the body. Without adequate protein your muscles weaken and your immune system becomes less effective. Protein is not stored, we need to consume it each day. Children need protein in their diet.

Do you find that your child is hungry right after a meal?

Then your child did not receive enough protein at the last meal.

Meat is not the only source of protein. Tofu is a great substitute for meat.

I use soy hot dogs and veggie burgers all the time. Most mainstream grocery stores carry these items.

Protein Choices

Skinless chicken
Turkey
Fish
Beef
Tofu
Milk
Cheese
Beans
Peas

Soybeans
Peanuts
Duck
Pork
Bacon
Deli meat
Lamb
Venison
Wild game
Buffalo

Carbohydrates

Carbohydrates are the pre-ferred energy food of the body.

You have to balance your car-bohydrate intake with your protein intake for your body to function properly. Carbohy-drates are not just grains, sweets and pasta; they also include fruits and vegetables.

Carbohydrate choices

Fruit
Vegetables
Bagels
Bread
Cereal
Grains
Rice
Pasta
Granola
bars

Pizza
Cookies
French fries
French
toast
Oatmeal
Muffins
Pancakes
Crackers

Fats

Fat is needed by the body, especially "good" fat. Mono-unsaturated fats come from nuts, avocados and olive oil. Omega-3 fats come from fish and fish oils.

All the other fats are considered "bad" fats. Your body can not properly absorb the "bad" fat. Processed foods contain bad fat!!!

Good fats

- Olive oil

- Nuts

- Avocados

- Fish

Bad fats

- Organ meat

- Fatty Red meat

- Processed Foods

- Oil used for frying
  in most restaurants

Do you know that your body needs fat to get rid of fat in your body?

Putting it all together

The body processes three major nutritional components:

Proteins, carbohydrates and fats. Now we will look at how it all works. Try feeding your child a snack when he or she is misbehaving and upset to see if she or he will calm down and become attentive. Try giving your child a bag of chips and a soda or fruit drink. Does the behavior change?

Most likely it will not. Your child will probably be more hungry and irritable than before.

This is because the child is not receiving what his or her body needs to sustain, grow and develop to his or her best abilities.

The result is an irritable, inattentive, difficult to manage child with frequent illnesses and difficulties in school.

OK then, let's briefly go over how the body uses protein, carbohydrates and fat.

All three play a major role in balancing the body's nutritional needs; each one has a unique effect.

Ready? ☺

Protein stimulates the release of glucagons which tell the body to release stored carbohydrates and replenish blood sugar levels for the brain. Without adequate glucagons you will always feel hungry and mentally tired because your brain is not getting enough of its primary fuel: blood sugar.

Carbohydrates stimulate insulin production, and insulin tells the body to store incoming nutrients.

As you can see, the more carbohydrates you eat the more insulin your body produces. Insulin and glucagons are performing a constant balancing act.

If one hormone goes up in the body the other one goes down.

Fat is needed for energy, and furthermore provides structure for the brain and all nerve tissues. Fat is by far the most important storage of fuel we have.

Your child will give you the clue!

Is he or she low on protein? Does your child have mood swings, decrease metal focus and is always hungry? Your child is eating too many carbohydrates and not enough protein.

Let's look at an average food intake of one day in an American child's life:

Breakfast : cereal with milk

Snack: granola bar

Lunch: Slice of pepperoni pizza, chocolate milk, orange

Snack: chips, cookies, soda

Dinner: Fast food Hamburger, French-fries, strawberry milk shake

Snack: Ice cream or candy bar

What is wrong with this picture?

The diet:

- Is high in *carbohydrates*, which are: Cereal, granola, pizza, chips, cookies, French fries, hamburger bun, and ice cream

- Contains *salicylate*s: Oranges, strawberry, tomato sauce

- Uses processed *milk products*: milk, milk shake, ice cream

- Contains *bad fats*: French fries, hamburger. Contains *TBHQ preservative*, which is added to the frying oil.

Let's change the menu to a healthier version and compare:

Breakfast: Cereal or oatmeal with two slices of bacon and water or juice to drink

Snack: Balanced nutritional bar or peanut butter crackers

Lunch: Turkey and cheese sandwich, cut cantaloupe and organic cheese puffs

Snack: Celery or banana with organic peanut butter

Dinner: Homemade chicken noodle soup with grilled cheese sandwich and fresh watermelon

Snack: Lemon-lime Popsicle

Do you see the difference?

Adjust your meals and your child will feel so much better. Try to use fresh, raw vegetables and fruit.

You have to provide balanced meals and snacks by balancing the carbohydrates and protein at each meal. Doing so will optimize the chance for your child to have a healthy happy day ☺ and be able to concentrate and mentally focus.

Wow!!! This was a challenging section.

I believe, that if you know the basics of the body's function you will be aware of the implications if giving your child a bag of chips or cookies. You will realize that you are throwing his or her body into overdrive while nutritionally depriving your child of the nutrients she or he needs.

On top of the protein-carbohydrate balancing act, your child's body must rid itself of all the chemicals, dyes, colorings in food.

A lot of work for such a little body. Don't you think?

Let's try to make things easier for your child and in return also for you. ☺

What kind of meals should I prepare?

Breakfast

- Oatmeal
- Bacon
- Waffles, syrup
- Sausage
- Bagels and cream cheese
- Shake with fruit
- Eggs (boiled, poached, scrambled)
- French toast
- Pancakes
- Cream of Wheat
- Toast with honey, cinnamon
- Hot chocolate milk

Check labels to ensure it is organic chocolate mix, organic cereal.

Remember to have Protein and Carbohydrates with each meal. This will optimize your child's brainpower. ☺

Snacks

- Deviled eggs
- Turkey
- Cheese and crackers
- Mustard as a dip
- Celery and peanut butter
- Peanut butter and jelly sandwich
- Peanut butter and honey sandwich
- Peanut butter, honey and banana sandwich
- Grilled cheese sandwich
- Nuts and seeds
- Popcorn with cheese
- Organic vanilla yoghurt and organic granola
- Soup and sandwich

Lunch

- leftover dinner
- hard boiled eggs
- organic dried turkey jerky
- Sandwich: turkey, cheese, peanut butter and jelly/honey
- Soup
- Salad with grilled chicken
- Fruit, nuts, veggies
- Chips, popcorn
- Organic cheese puffs
- Grilled cheese sandwich
- Soup and sandwich

Invest in a thermos. If you pour hot water in the thermos prior to filling it up with the food, it will keep the food hot until lunch.

☺ Most children love this idea!

Basic Recipe Ideas for Snacks

Yellow Cake

¾ cup milk
1 ½ cup sugar
3 eggs
4 ½ tsp baking powder
½ tsp salt
3 cups cake flour or
2 2/3 cups of regular flour
1 cup milk
1 ½ tsp vanilla (pure vanilla)
Creamed butter and sugar.

Add eggs. Beat mixture until smooth. Add baking powder, salt, vanilla. Beat just to blend.

Add ½ cup of flour at a time, then a little bit of milk; repeat until all is mixed in.

Bake at 375 degrees for 25 min to 30 min.

For chocolate cake:

Add 3 tbs. of cocoa or 1½ blocks of chocolate melted.

Butter Frosting

6 tbs. Butter
1 16-oz pkg. powder sugar
4 Tbs. milk
1 ½ tsp vanilla

Mix butter until light and fluffy

Gradually add half of the sugar, then beat in 2 tbs. milk and vanilla. Gradually add remaining powdered sugar, beating constantly. Add 2 more tbs. to make frosting a smooth consistency.

The natural way to add color
to food ☺

- **Yellow**: add turmeric

- **Pink**: chop beets and
  cook them in a small
  amount of water.

- **Red**: Concentrated beet
  juice. Freeze frosting for
  two days to deepen
  color.

- **Purple**: Boil red cabbage. Freeze frosting for
  two days to deepen
  color.

- **Green**: Cook chopped
  spinach only to a bright
  green stage. Puree in
  blender using small
  amounts of frosting.
  Keep in freezer. This
  color will have green
  specks.

- **Blue**: Add baking soda
  to the cabbage juice

- **Brown**: Add cocoa to
  some of the frosting

Chocolate Frosting

4Tbs softened butter
2 cups powdered sugar
½ cup cocoa
dash of salt
1 tsp vanilla
¼ cup milk

Mix ingredients except milk. Then add 2 tbs. of milk at a time to reach desired consistency.

Ginger Snaps

(Without cloves; remember, cloves are a salicylate)

1 egg beaten
1 cup sugar
¾ cup shortening
¼ cup molasses
½ tsp cinnamon
½ tsp ground ginger
2 ½ tsp baking soda
pinch of salt
2 cups flour

Mix all ingredients except sugar. Form a 1 inch ball. Roll in sugar. Bake for 10 minutes on an ungreased cookie sheet. Makes four dozen.

Peanut Butter Cups

1 package of bittersweet
chocolate
Organic peanut butter
Small cupcake forms

Melt chocolate. Microwave
until smooth (be careful not to
let chocolate burn) or melt
slowly on stove. Use larger pot
half filled with water and set
glass bowl with chocolate into
the warm water. Pour 1 tsp.
of melted chocolate into cup.
Push chocolate up on the
sides of cup. Wait ten minutes
until firm consistency or place
in refrigerator for quicker results.

Add ½ tsp. peanut butter into
the middle; add ½ tsp. melted
chocolate to cover peanut butter.

Place in refrigerator to chill.

Lemon Ice Cream

1 c. milk (organic is preferred)
1 c. half and half
1 c. sweetened condensed
milk

⅜ c. lemon juice
¾ tsp lemon grind
¼ c sugar

Beat all ingredients together

Freeze

Homemade Frozen Juice Treat

Pour Mango, Papaya or Pear juice into a plastic cup and freeze. Kids love to scrape the frozen juice out of the cup as an evening snack.

Substitute, do not deprive ☺

Halloween

Please, allow your child to participate in the tradition. You can have the Halloween Fairy come to your house.

The "Halloween Fairy" comes the night after Halloween. Your child places the bucket of candy at the front door and then in the morning the Halloween Fairy exchanges the candy for a great toy.

Many children just love this idea and they are happy with just getting a few pieces of candy. Older children enjoy this idea too especially if they receive money the next morning.

Check your candy to make sure they don't contain any food dyes or coloring. Chocolate candy bars are your best choice. Focus most of your energy on the costume and decorating pumpkins.

Enjoy the excitement of your child. Include the *BECLL Ap-*

proach; boundaries, empathy, consistency, love and laughter. ☺

Conclusion

A Note from the Author

My hope is that my book will assist you in making positive changes in your life, and also to provide you with alternatives and hope. No matter what the past was like for you, it is never too late to change.

You can always start today.

I believe that most of our children have vivid imaginations. In time, with kindness and patience, you will be able to see the positive sides of your very emotional child.

You will learn to appreciate his or her strength and move forward.

Conclusion

I would like to leave you with a phrase I came across; the author is unknown.

It is quite possible

to successfully raise

a difficult child.

All it requires is

that you are

twice as good at it

as most other parents.

Conclusion

Membership information

Feingold Association

www.feingold.org

1.800.321.3287

P.O. Box 6550

Alexandria, VA. 22306

This organization will provide you with updated particular food lists acceptable to your region of the USA. Feingold Association has researched thousand of name brand items free of unwanted additives. You can fine tune the information I provided to you.

Feingold Association will do the work for you and you can ask for specific food items to be researched for free. With a one-time membership fee of around seventy dollars you will receive:

Food lists, Feingold handbook, medication list, recipes, and "Pure Fact," which is a newsletter updating you to

Conclusion

which brand name foods to remove or to add.

I am also a member and find the information extremely helpful.

Conclusion

About the Author

Dr. Cathrin Olsen holds a Doctorate in Naturology and is a member of the American Alternative Medical Association.

Her background in the medical field as a Registered Nurse has provided her with extensive experience, contributing to her well rounded knowledge both in the holistic and medical field.

Dr. Olsen's initial career years took her through the demanding work within the psychiatric and chemical dependency field. The years following she spent as a home health nurse specializing in infusion therapy, providing chemotherapy, antibiotic therapy as well as total nutritional therapy to patients. She then turned her attention to assessing psychiatric patients in their homes and concentrated on being a liaison for Hospice, working with dying patients as well as their families.

Conclusion

Throughout her career as a Registered Nurse, Dr. Olsen noticed an immense correlation between food intake, physical ailment and behavior. Her real challenge came as her youngest child had enormous difficulties coping with everyday life.

After receiving her doctorate, she decided to dedicate herself to researching alternative options for ADD, ADHD and Ritalin use.

Dr. Olsen's extensive research in the USA, as well as in Europe, especially Germany, has reiterated her findings about the distinct correlation between food intake, physical ailments and behavioral patterns.

Her determination and diligent work has cumulated in a delightful and very informative book *"Is this really my child?"*

Conclusion

She focuses on "temperamentally difficult" children and provides a refreshing innovative approach as well as profound assistance to parents dealing with their children.

Dr. Olsen does not believe in labeling children as ADD and ADHD, as a result referring to these children as "temperamentally difficult".

Over the years she has volunteered her time for the battered wife shelter, women's health groups, parent-teacher associations, youth organizations and as a family liaison for the U.S. Navy.

Dr. Olsen lives in Coronado, California, with her husband, five children, and their Golden Retriever.

Further Information and assistance

If you need further assistance and help, feel free to contact me.

I'm available to you through email. I truly want you to be a pleased parent with a happy child.

www.ADDnoMore.com

DrOlsenC@ADDnomore.com

Sincerely,

Dr. Cathrin Olsen